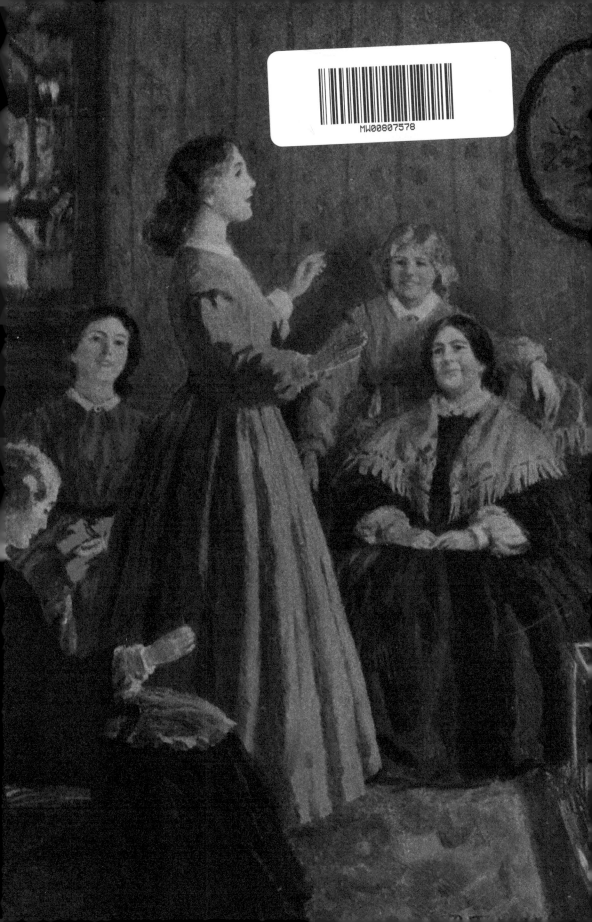

A Dovetale Press Adaptation

Little Women

Louisa May Alcott

Adaptation by
Dr Gillian Claridge
Dr B. Sally Rimkeit

Illustrations by
Clara M Burd
Harold Copping
Percy Tarrant

A Dovetale Press Adaptation
Little Women
Louisa May Alcott

Adapted by Dr Gillian Claridge and Dr B. Sally Rimkeit
Copyright 2016 © Gillian Claridge and B. Sally Rimkeit

All original material in Public Domain
Illustration scans from Dovetale Press private collections
Original Text from Project Gutenberg

This edition published by Dovetale Press 2016

National Library of New Zealand Cataloguing-in-Publication Data:
Claridge, Gillian
A Dovetale Press Adaptation, Little Women Louisa May Alcott/
adaptation by Dr Gillian Claridge and Dr B. Sally Rimkeit;
original text from Project Gutenberg.
ISBN 978-0-473-37295-8
I. Rimkeit, Sally, 1958- II. Alcott, Louisa May, 1832-1888.
Little Women.
III. Title.
NZ823.3—dc 23

Comments and questions, please email: editor@dovetalepress.com

All titles in this Dovetale Press series are carefully constructed to enhance
readability. Our other titles are
A Dovetale Books Adaptation of A Christmas Carol by Charles Dickens
ISBN 978-0-473-37294-1
A Dovetale Press Adaptation of The Garden Party & The Doll's House
by Katherine Mansfield ISBN 978-0-473-37291-0
A Dovetale Press Adaptation of Sherlock Holmes: The Adventure of the
Blue Carbuncle by Arthur Conan Doyle ISBN 978-0-473-37293-4
A Dovetale Press Selection: Poetry for the Restless Heart
ISBN 978-0-473-37292-7

CONTENTS

CAST OF CHARACTERS

Meg March: Sixteen years old and the eldest March sister, very pretty.

Jo March: Fifteen years old, tall, thin and brown, with big hands and feet.

Beth March: Thirteen years old, rosy, smooth-haired, bright-eyed, with a shy manner, a timid voice, and a peaceful expression.

Amy March: The youngest sister, with blue eyes, and yellow hair curling on her shoulders, pale and slender, rather spoiled.

Mrs March: Mother of Meg, Jo, Beth and Amy, who call her Marmee.

Mr March: An army chaplain for the Union troops fighting the American Civil War.

Hannah: The faithful servant to the Marches.

Aunt March: Mr March's elderly rich aunt, who is fond of the family but despises Mr March's inability to make money.

Laurie, the Laurence boy: Sixteen years old, an orphan who lives with his grandfather next door to the Marches.

Mr Laurence: The wealthy, crusty old man who lives next door to the Marches and is grandfather to Laurie.

John Brooke: Laurie's tutor, in love with Meg.

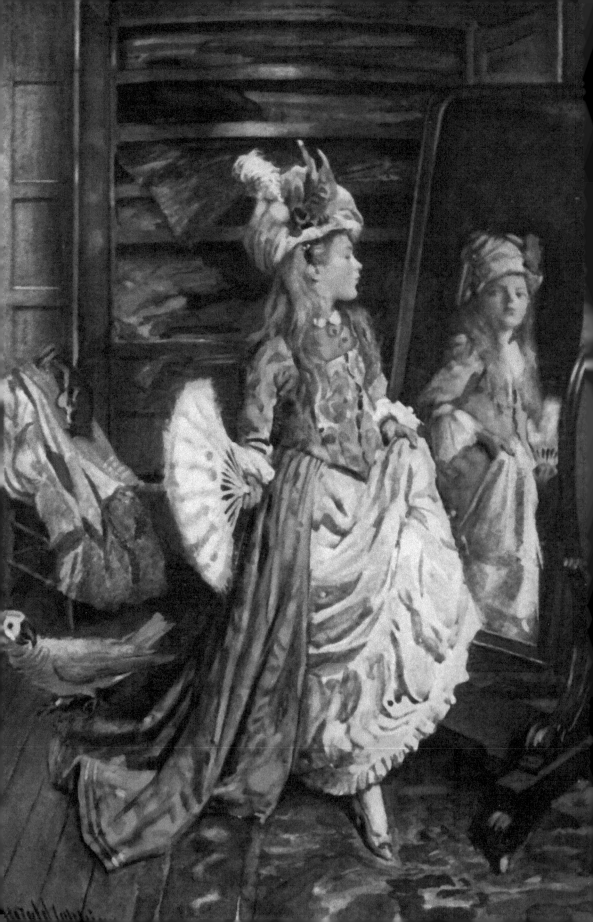

CHAPTER 1: A MERRY CHRISTMAS

"Christmas won't be Christmas without any presents," grumbled Jo, lying on the rug.

"It's so dreadful to be poor!" sighed Meg, looking down at her old dress.

"I don't think it's fair for some girls to have plenty of pretty things, and other girls nothing at all," added little Amy, with an injured sniff.

"We've got Father and Mother, and each other," said Beth contentedly from her corner.

The four young faces on which the firelight shone brightened at the cheerful words, but darkened again as Jo said sadly, "We haven't got Father, and shall not have him for a long time."

The clock struck six and, having swept up the hearth, Beth put a pair of slippers down to warm. Somehow the sight of the old shoes had a good effect upon the girls, for Marmee was coming, and everyone brightened to welcome her.

Jo forgot how tired she was as she sat up to hold the slippers nearer to the blaze.

"They are quite worn out. Marmee must have a new pair," she said.

"I'll tell you what we'll do," said Beth. "Let's each get her something for Christmas, and not get anything for ourselves."

"That's like you, dear! I shall get her army slippers, best to be had," cried Jo.

Meg announced, "I shall give her a nice pair of gloves."

"Some handkerchiefs, all hemmed," said Beth.

"I'll get a little bottle of cologne. She likes it, and it won't cost much, so I'll have some left to buy my pencils," added Amy.

Jo was the first to wake in the gray dawn of Christmas morning. No stockings hung at the fireplace. For a moment she felt as much disappointed as she did long ago, when her little sock fell down because it was crammed so full of goodies.

But her mother had promised that there would be one present for each of the sisters. And under each of their pillows was a little book, the beautiful story of the best life ever lived. In each book Marmee had written a few words, which made their one gift very precious in their eyes.

"Where is Marmee?" asked Meg, as she and Jo ran down to thank her for their gifts half an hour later.

"Goodness only knows. Some poor creeter came a-beggin', and your ma went straight off to see what was needed. There never was such a woman for givin' away vittles and drink, clothes and firin'," replied Hannah. She had lived with the family since Meg was born, and was considered by them all more as a friend than a servant.

Amy came in hastily and looked rather abashed when she saw her sisters all waiting for her.

"Where have you been and what are you hiding behind you?" asked Meg. She was surprised to see by her hood and cloak that lazy Amy had been out so early.

"Don't laugh at me!" said Amy. "I only meant to change the little bottle of cologne for a big one, and I gave all my money to get it. I'm truly trying not to be selfish anymore." Amy looked so earnest and humble in her little effort to forget herself that Meg hugged her on the spot.

The door banged again, and the girls rushed to greet their mother.

"Merry Christmas, Marmee! Many of them! Thank you for our books. We read some, and mean to every day," they all cried in chorus.

"Merry Christmas, little daughters!

"But I want to say one word before we sit down.

"Not far away from here lies a poor German woman with a little newborn baby. Six children are huddled into one bed to keep from freezing, for they have no fire. There is nothing to eat over there, and the oldest boy came to tell me they were suffering hunger and cold. My girls, will you give the Hummels your breakfast as a Christmas present?"

For a minute no one spoke, and then Jo exclaimed impetuously, "I'm so glad you came before we began!"

Mrs March smiled. "You shall all go and help me take breakfast to the Hummels, and when we come back we will have bread and milk, and make it up at dinnertime."

They were soon ready, and the procession set out.

A poor, bare, miserable room it was, with broken windows, no fire, ragged bedclothes, a sick mother, wailing baby, and a group of pale, hungry children cuddled under one old quilt, trying to keep warm.

How the big eyes stared and the blue lips smiled as the girls went in.

"Ach ein Gott! Die engel-kinder. It is child angels come to us!" said the poor woman, crying for joy, "Oh my God."

"Funny angels in hoods and mittens," said Jo, and set them to laughing.

Hannah, who had carried wood, made the fire. Mrs March gave the mother tea and gruel. The girls meantime spread the table, set the children round the fire, and fed them like so many hungry birds, laughing and talking.

"Das ist gut! Die engel-kinder!" cried the poor children as they ate and warmed their purple hands at the comfortable blaze, "This is good."

The girls had never been called angel children before and thought it very agreeable. That was a very happy breakfast, though they didn't get any of it.

Back home, they set out their presents while their mother was upstairs collecting clothes for the poor Hummels. When she came down, Mrs March was both surprised and touched. She smiled with her eyes full as she examined her presents and read the little notes which accompanied them.

The morning charities and ceremonies took so much time that the rest of the day was devoted to preparations for the evening festivities. Not being rich enough to go often to the theater, the girls played in their own theatrical productions, written by Jo.

No gentlemen were admitted, so Jo played male parts to her heart's content. She took immense satisfaction in a pair of russet leather boots given her by a friend, who knew a lady who knew an actor.

On Christmas night, a dozen girls piled onto the bed which was the dress circle. They sat before the blue and yellow chintz curtains in a most flattering state of expectancy.

There was a good deal of rustling and whispering behind the curtains, a trifle of lamp smoke, and an occasional giggle from Amy, who was apt to get hysterical in the excitement of the moment.

The opera was a splendid creation, in which Jo played both villain Hugo and hero Rodrigo, wearing the boots for both parts. Shy Beth played servants and jailers. It concluded with the witch Hagar, played by Meg, poisoning the villain Hugo. Zara, played by Amy, and Rodrigo were then free to marry. So all ended happily.

Tumultuous applause followed the performance but received an unexpected check. The cot bed, on which the dress circle was built, suddenly shut up and extinguished the enthusiastic audience.
Jo and Meg flew to the rescue. All were taken out unhurt, though many were speechless with laughter.

The excitement had hardly subsided when Hannah appeared with Mrs March's compliments, saying "would the ladies walk down to supper."

When the actors saw the supper table, they looked at one another in rapturous amazement. There was ice cream, actually two dishes of it, pink and white, and cake and fruit, and distracting French bonbons. In the middle of the table were four great bouquets of hot house flowers.

It quite took their breath away, and they stared first at the table and then at their mother.

"Is it fairies?" asked Amy.

"Santa Claus," said Beth.

"Marmee did it." And Meg smiled her sweetest.

"Aunt March had a good fit and sent the supper," cried Jo, with a sudden inspiration.

"All wrong. Old Mr Laurence sent it," replied Mrs March.

"The Laurence boy's grandfather! What in the world put such a thing into his head? We don't know him!" exclaimed Meg.

"Hannah told one of his servants about your breakfast party," said Mrs March. "He is an odd old gentleman, but that pleased him. So you have a little feast at night to make up for the bread-and-milk breakfast."

"That boy put it into his head, I know he did! He's a capital fellow, and I wish we could get acquainted," said Jo.

Mrs March said, "I like the boy's manners, so I've no objection to your knowing him. He brought the flowers himself. I should have asked him in, if I had been sure what was going on upstairs. He looked so wistful as he went away, hearing the frolic and evidently having none of his own."

"It's a mercy you didn't, Marmee!" laughed Jo, looking at her boots. "But we'll have another play sometime that he can see. Perhaps he'll help act. Wouldn't that be jolly?"

"I never had such a fine bouquet before! How pretty it is!" And Meg examined her flowers with great interest.

But Beth whispered softly, "I wish I could send my bunch to Father. I'm afraid he isn't having such a merry Christmas as we are."

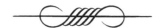

A MERRY CHRISTMAS:
CHAPTER SUMMARY

We meet Meg, Jo, Beth and Amy, the March sisters. They give away their Christmas breakfast and entertain their friends with an operatic performance written by Jo.

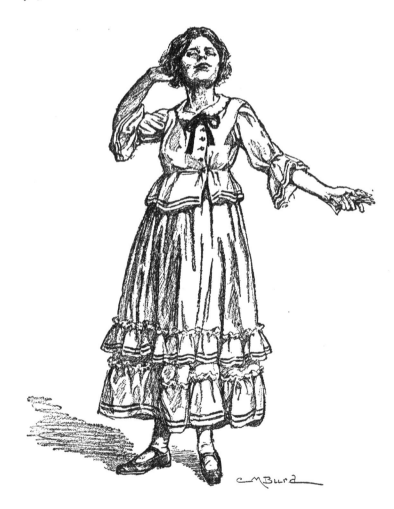

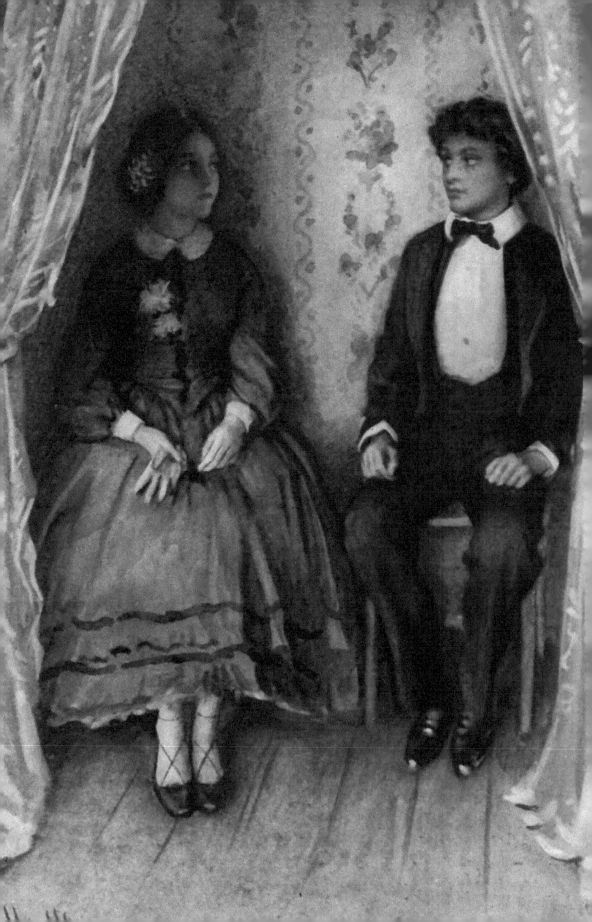

CHAPTER 2: THE LAURENCE BOY

"Jo! Jo! Where are you?" cried Meg at the foot of the garret stairs.

"Here!" answered a husky voice from above. Running up, Meg found her sister eating apples and crying over a romantic novel.

"Such fun! Only see! An invitation!" cried Meg, waving the precious paper. She read out, "'Mrs Gardiner would be happy to see Miss March and Miss Josephine at a little dance on New Year's Eve.' Marmee is willing we should go, now what shall we wear?"

"Your poplin dress is as good as new, but there is that burn and a tear in mine," said Jo, who never troubled herself much about dress. "Whatever shall I do?"

"Jo, you must sit still all you can and keep your back out of sight," advised Meg. "The front is all right. And do behave nicely! Don't put your hands behind you, or stare, or say 'Christopher Columbus!' will you?"

"Don't worry about me. I'll be as prim as I can and not get into any scrapes, if I can help it," said Jo. "Now go and accept the invitation, and let me finish this splendid story."

On New Year's Eve, the whole family was absorbed in the all-important business of preparing for the party. At last both girls were ready. Meg's high-heeled slippers were very tight and hurt her. Jo's nineteen hairpins all seemed stuck straight into her head, which was not exactly comfortable. But, dear me, let us be elegant or die.

Hannah walked them to Mrs Gardiner's house. They entered feeling a trifle timid, for they seldom went to parties, and this little gathering was an event to them.

Mrs Gardiner, a stately old lady, greeted them kindly and handed them over to Sallie, her daughter. Meg knew Sallie and was at her ease very soon. But Jo, who didn't care much for girls or girlish gossip, stood about, with her back carefully against the wall. She felt as much out of place as a colt in a flower garden.

Jo could not roam about and amuse herself, for the burned part of her dress would show. So she slipped into a curtained recess, intending to peep at the dancing and enjoy herself in peace.

Unfortunately, another bashful person had chosen the same refuge. As the curtain fell behind her, she found herself face to face with the Laurence boy, their neighbor who had once brought their lost cat home.

"Dear me, I didn't know anyone was here!" stammered Jo, preparing to back out as speedily as she had bounced in.

The Laurence boy laughed and said pleasantly, though he looked a little startled, "Don't mind me. Stay if you like."

He sat down and looked at his shoes, till Jo said, trying to be polite and easy, "I think I've had the pleasure of seeing you before. You live near us, don't you?"

"Next door." And he looked up and laughed outright, for Jo's prim manner was rather funny when he remembered how they had chatted about cricket when he had brought the cat home.

So, trying to look sober, while his black eyes shone with fun, he asked, "How is your cat, Miss March?"

"Nicely, thank you, Mr Laurence. But I am not Miss March, I'm only Jo," returned the young lady.

"I'm not Mr Laurence. I'm only Laurie."

"Laurie Laurence, what an odd name," said Jo.

"My first name is Theodore, but I don't like it, for the fellows called me Dora so I made them say Laurie instead."

"I hate my name, too, so sentimental! I wish every one would say Jo instead of Josephine. How did you make the boys stop calling you Dora?"

"I thrashed 'em."

"I can't thrash Aunt March, so I suppose I shall have to bear it," sighed Jo with resignation.

Both were soon chatting till they felt like old acquaintances. Laurie's bashfulness soon wore off, for Jo's gentlemanly demeanor amused and set him at his ease. And Jo was her merry self again, because her dress was forgotten.

"Don't you like to dance, Miss Jo?" asked Laurie, looking as if he thought the name suited her.

"I like to dance well enough if there is plenty of room, and everyone is lively. In a place like this I'm sure to tread on people's toes, so I keep out of mischief and let Meg sail about. Listen, they're playing a splendid polka! Why don't you go and try it?" said Jo.

"If you will come too," Laurie answered with a gallant little bow.

"I can't, for I told Meg I wouldn't, because…" There Jo stopped, and looked undecided whether to tell or to laugh.

"Because, what?" asked Laurie kindly.

"Because…I've scorched my dress and Meg told me to keep still so no one would see it. You may laugh, if you want to. It is funny, I know."

Laurie didn't laugh. He only looked down a minute and said very gently, "Never mind that. I'll tell you how we can manage. There's a long empty hall out there, and we can dance grandly, and no one will see us. Please come."

Jo thanked him, and they had a grand polka, for Laurie danced well. They were sitting on the stairs afterwards when Meg appeared and beckoned Jo into a side room.

There Meg collapsed on a sofa, holding her foot and looking pale.

"I've sprained my ankle. That stupid high heel turned. It aches so. I can hardly stand, and I don't know how I'm ever going to get home," Meg said, rocking to and fro in pain.

"I don't see what we can do, except get a carriage," said Jo.

"It will cost ever so much, and I dare say I can't get one at all, for there is no one to send for it. I will wait here until Hannah comes to take us home, though I don't know how I will walk. Would you run along and get me some coffee? I'm so tired I can't stir."

Jo found the dining room and, making a dive at the table, she secured the coffee. Colliding with another guest, she immediately spilled it, thereby making the front of her dress as bad as the back.

"Can I help you?" said a friendly voice. And there was Laurie, with a full cup in one hand and a plate of ice cream in the other.

"I was trying to get something for Meg, who is very tired, and some one shook me. Here I am in a nice state," answered Jo, looking at the coffee on her dress.

"Too bad! I was looking for someone to give this coffee to. May I take it to your sister?" asked Laurie.

"Oh, thank you! I'll show you where she is," and Jo led the way. As if used to waiting on ladies, Laurie drew up a little table and brought a second installment of coffee and ice cream for Jo. He was so obliging that even particular Meg pronounced him a "nice boy."

When Hannah arrived, Meg stood up and was forced to catch hold of Jo, with an exclamation of pain. Hannah scolded, Meg cried, and Jo decided to go and find a carriage, but there were none. She was looking round for help when Laurie offered his grandfather's carriage, which had just come for him.

"It's so early! You can't mean to go yet?" began Jo, looking relieved but hesitating to accept the offer.

"I always go early, I do, truly! Please let me take you home. It's all on my way, you know, and it may rain," Laurie offered.

That settled it, and telling Laurie of Meg's mishap, Jo gratefully accepted. Hannah hated rain as much as a cat does, so she made no trouble. They rolled away in the luxurious closed carriage, feeling very festive and elegant.

"I declare, it really seems like being a fine young lady, to come home from the party in a carriage and sit in my dressing gown with a maid to wait on me," said Meg later in their bedroom, as Jo bound up her foot with arnica and brushed her hair.

"In spite of our burned gowns, and tight slippers that sprain our ankles when we are silly enough to wear them, I don't believe young ladies enjoy themselves any more than we do," exclaimed Jo.

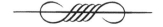

THE LAURENCE BOY:
CHAPTER SUMMARY

Meg and Jo are invited to a New Year's party.
Jo has difficulty with her dress, and meets Laurie,
the Laurence boy who lives next door to them.
Meg sprains her ankle, and Laurie takes them home
in the Laurence carriage.

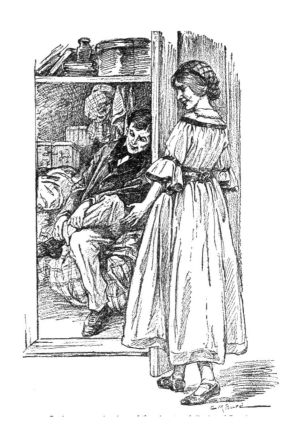

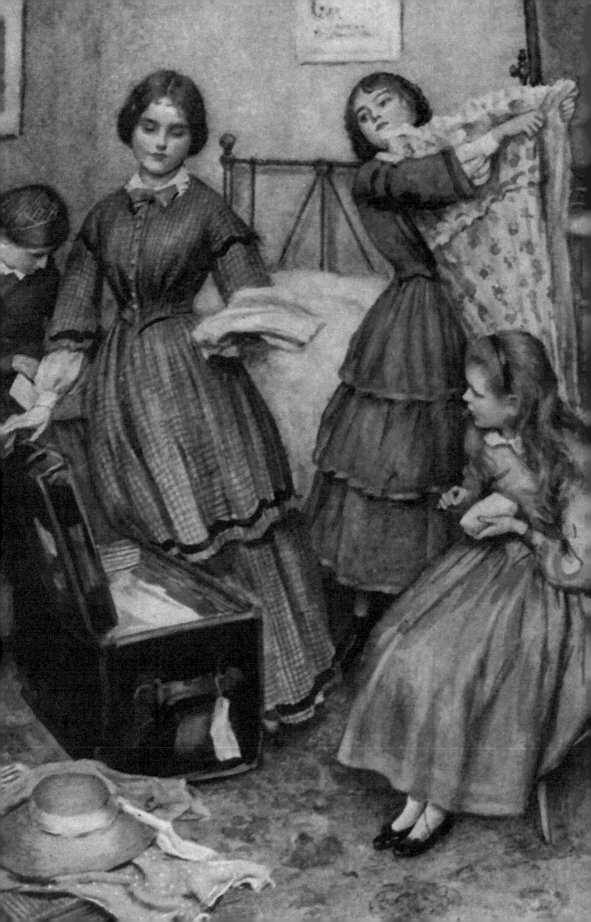

CHAPTER 3: JO'S ANGRY DEMON

"Jo and Meg, where are you going?" asked Amy, coming into their room one Saturday afternoon, and finding them getting ready to go out with an air of secrecy which excited her curiosity.

"I know! I know! You're going to the theater to see the 'Seven Castles!' she cried, adding resolutely, "and I shall go too, for Marmee said I might see it, and I've got my rag money, and it was mean not to tell me in time."

"Just listen to me a minute, and be a good child," said Meg soothingly. "Marmee doesn't wish you to go this week, because you have a nasty cold. Next week you can go with Beth and Hannah, and have a nice time."

"I don't like that half as well as going with you and Laurie. Please let me. I've been sick with this cold so long and shut up. I'm dying for some fun. Do, Meg! I'll be ever so good," pleaded Amy, looking as pathetic as she could.

But Jo said, "You can't sit with us, for our seats are reserved. You mustn't sit alone, for Laurie will give you his place, and that will spoil our pleasure. Or he'll get another seat for you, and that isn't proper when you weren't asked. You shan't stir a step, so you may just stay where you are."

Laurie called from below. The two girls hurried down, leaving Amy wailing, for now and then she forgot her grown-up ways and acted like a spoiled child.

Just as the party was setting out, Amy called over the banisters in a threatening tone, "You'll be sorry for this, Jo March, see if you ain't."

"Fiddlesticks!" returned Jo, slamming the door.

They had a charming time, for "The Seven Castles Of The Diamond Lake" was as brilliant and wonderful as the heart could wish.

When they got home, they found Amy reading in the parlor. She assumed an injured air as they came in, and never lifted her eyes from her book. Jo decided that Amy had forgiven and forgotten her wrongs.

There Jo was mistaken, for next day she made a discovery which produced a tempest.

Meg, Beth, and Amy were sitting together, late in the afternoon, when Jo burst into the room, looking excited and demanding breathlessly, "Has anyone taken my book?"

Meg and Beth said, "No" at once, and looked surprised. Amy poked the fire and said nothing.

Jo saw her color rise and was down upon her in a minute. "Amy, you've got it!"

"No, I haven't," said Amy.

"You know where it is, then!"cried Jo.

"No, I don't," said Amy.

"That's a fib!" Jo cried. "You know something about it, and you'd better tell at once, or I'll make you."

"Scold as much as you like. You'll never see your silly old book again," cried Amy, getting excited in her turn.

"Why not?" Jo asked.

"I burned it up!" said Amy.

"What! My little book of fairy tales I worked so hard on, and meant to finish before Father got home? Have you really burned it?" said Jo, her eyes kindling.

"Yes, I did! I told you I'd make you pay for being so cross yesterday, and I have, so…"

"You wicked, wicked girl! I never can write it again, and I'll never forgive you as long as I live."

When Mrs March came home and heard the story, she soon brought Amy to a sense of the wrong she had done her sister.

As Jo received her good-night kiss, Mrs March whispered gently, "My dear, don't let the sun go down upon your anger."

But Jo shook her head and said gruffly, because Amy was listening, "It was an abominable thing, and she doesn't deserve to be forgiven."

Next day, Jo still looked like a thunder cloud, and nothing went well all day.

"Everybody is so hateful, I'll ask Laurie to go skating," said Jo to herself. "He is always kind and jolly, and will put me to rights, I know," and off she went.

Amy heard the clash of skates, and looked out with an impatient exclamation.

"There! Jo promised I should go next time, for this is the last ice we shall have. But it's no use to ask such a crosspatch to take me," Amy said to Meg.

"Don't say that. You were very naughty, and it is hard to forgive the loss of her precious little book. But I think she might do it now, if you try her at the right minute," said Meg. "Go after them and when she seems to be feeling more good natured, just kiss her and show you are sorry."

"I'll try," said Amy, and she ran after the friends, who were just disappearing over the hill.
When they got to the river, Jo saw her coming, and turned her back.

Laurie did not see, for he was carefully skating along the shore, sounding the ice, because a warm spell had preceded the cold snap. "I'll go on to the first bend and see if it's all right before we begin to race," Amy heard him say. But she did not hear him say to Jo, "Keep near the shore. It isn't safe in the middle."

Jo glanced over her shoulder. The angry little demon she was harboring said in her ear, "No matter whether Amy heard or not, let her take care of herself."

Laurie had vanished round the bend and Jo was just at the turn. Amy was far behind, striking out toward the smoother ice in the middle of the river.

For a minute Jo stood still with a strange feeling in her heart. She resolved to go on, but something held and turned her round. She saw Amy throw up her hands and go down, with a sudden crash of rotten ice, the splash of water, and a cry that made Jo's heart stand still with fear.

Jo tried to call Laurie, but her voice was gone. She tried to rush forward, but her feet seemed to have no strength in them. For a second, she could only stand motionless, staring with a terror-stricken face at Amy's little blue hood above the black water.

Something rushed swiftly by Jo, and Laurie's voice cried out, "Bring a rail. Quick, quick!" Together they got Amy out, more frightened than hurt.

"Now then, we must walk her home as fast as we can. Pile our things on her, while I get off these confounded skates," cried Laurie, wrapping his coat round Amy. He tugged away at the skate straps which never seemed so intricate before.

Shivering, dripping and crying, they got Amy home, who fell asleep rolled in blankets before a hot fire.

When the house was finally quiet, and Mrs March was sitting by the bed, Jo asked remorsefully, "Are you sure she is safe?"

"Quite safe, dear. She is not hurt, and won't even take cold, I think. You were so sensible in covering and getting her home quickly," replied her mother cheerfully.

"Laurie did it all. I only let her go. Marmee, if she should die, it would be my fault." And Jo dropped down beside the bed in a passion of penitent tears, telling all that had happened, bitterly condemning her hardness of heart.

"It's my dreadful temper! I try to cure it. I think I have, and then it breaks out worse than ever. Oh, Marmee, what shall I do? What shall I do?" cried poor Jo in despair.

"Watch and pray, dear. Never get tired of trying, and never think it is impossible to conquer your fault," said Mrs March. "You think your temper is the worst in the world, but mine used to be just like it."

"Yours, Marmee? Why, you are never angry!" And for the moment Jo forgot remorse in surprise.

"I've been trying to cure it for forty years, and have only succeeded in controlling it."

Jo felt comforted at once by the sympathy and confidence given her. The knowledge that her mother had a fault like hers and tried to mend it strengthened her resolution to cure it, though forty years seemed rather a long time to watch and pray to a girl of fifteen.

Amy stirred and sighed in her sleep. Eager to begin at once to mend her fault, Jo looked up with an expression on her face which it had never worn before.

"I let the sun go down on my anger. I wouldn't forgive her, and today, if it hadn't been for Laurie, it might have been too late! How could I be so wicked?" said Jo, half aloud, as she leaned over her sister, softly stroking the wet hair scattered on the pillow.

As if she heard, Amy opened her eyes, and held out her arms with a smile that went straight to Jo's heart. Neither said a word, but they hugged one another close, in spite of the blankets, and everything was forgiven and forgotten in one hearty kiss.

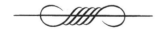

JO'S ANGRY DEMON:
CHAPTER SUMMARY

Amy is furious because she is not allowed to go to
the theatre with Meg, Jo and Laurie. Amy burns
Jo's precious book and so Jo is angry with her.
When Amy tries to go skating with Jo and Laurie,
Jo ignores her. Amy almost drowns by falling
through the ice, but Laurie saves her. Jo is very
sorry and asks her mother's help in controlling
her temper.

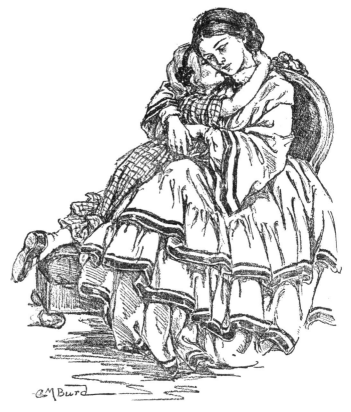

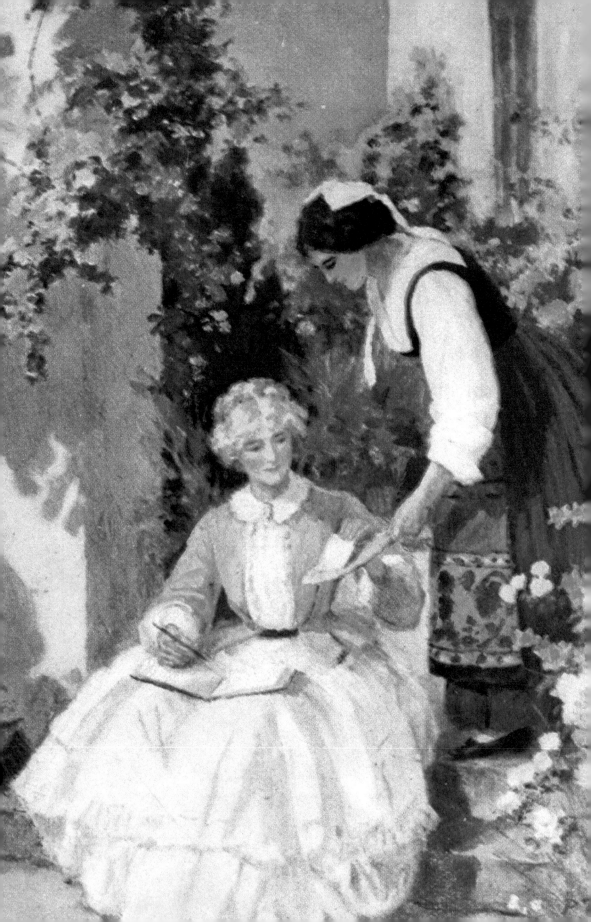

CHAPTER 4: A TELEGRAM

"November is the most disagreeable month in the whole year," said Meg, standing at the window one dull afternoon, looking out at the frostbitten garden.

"That's the reason I was born in it," observed Jo pensively, quite unconscious of the blot on her nose.

A sharp ring at the door interrupted them, and a minute after Hannah came in with a letter. "It's one of them horrid telegraph things, mum," she said, handing it to Mrs March as if she was afraid it would explode and do some damage.

At the word 'telegraph', Mrs March snatched it and read the two lines it contained. She dropped back into her chair as white as if the little paper had sent a bullet to her heart.

Jo read aloud, in a frightened voice:
"'Mrs March: Your husband is very ill. Come at once. S. HALE Blank Hospital, Washington.'"

How suddenly the whole world seemed to change. The girls gathered about their mother, feeling as if all the happiness and support of their lives was about to be taken from them.

For several minutes there was nothing but the sound of sobbing in the room, mingled with broken words of comfort.

Hannah was the first to recover, and exclaimed, "The Lord keep the dear man! I won't waste no time a-cryin', but git your things ready right away, mum," and she went away to work like three women in one.

Mrs March said, "She's right, there's no time for tears now. Be calm, girls. Laurie, would you please send a telegram saying I will take the next train and be there tomorrow."

Next day, in the cold gray dawn, the sisters lit their lamp. As they dressed, they agreed to send their mother on her anxious journey unsaddened by tears or complaints from them. Breakfast at that early hour seemed odd, and even Hannah's familiar face looked unnatural as she flew about her kitchen with her nightcap on.

Before their mother went none of the girls cried. No one ran away or uttered a lamentation, though their hearts were very heavy as they sent loving messages to Father.

But when Marmee had left, and in spite of their brave resolutions, they all broke down and cried bitterly.

During the next week, news from their father comforted the girls very much, for though dangerously ill, the presence of the best and tenderest of nurses had already done him good.

A bulletin was sent every day. As the head of the family, Meg insisted on reading the dispatches, which grew more cheerful as time passed.

For this first week the amount of virtue in the old house would have supplied the neighborhood. It was really amazing, for everyone seemed in a heavenly frame of mind, and self-denial was all the fashion. However, relieved of their first anxiety about their father, the girls insensibly relaxed their praiseworthy efforts a little.

The girls began to fall back into old ways, until one afternoon Beth said, "Meg, I wish you'd go and see the Hummels. You know Marmee told us not to forget them."

"Why don't you go yourself?" asked Meg.

"I have been every day, but the baby is sick.
I don't know what to do for it, so I think you or Hannah ought to go."

But no one else wanted to go. Beth quietly put on her hood and filled her basket with odds and ends for the poor children. She went out into the chilly air with a heavy head and a grieved look in her patient eyes. It was late when she came back. No one saw her creep upstairs and shut herself into her mother's room.

Half an hour after, Jo went to Marmee's closet for something. There she found little Beth sitting on the medicine chest, looking very grave, with red eyes and a camphor bottle in her hand.

"Christopher Columbus! What's the matter?" cried Jo.

Beth put out her hand as if to warn Jo off, and asked quickly, "You've had the scarlet fever, haven't you?"

"Years ago, when Meg did. Why?"

"Then I'll tell you. Oh, Jo, the baby's dead!"

"What baby?"

"Mrs Hummel's. It died in my lap before Mrs Hummel got home," cried Beth with a sob.

"Don't cry, dear! What did you do?"

"I just sat and held it softly till Mrs Hummel came with the doctor. He said it was dead, and looked at the other Hummel children, who have sore throats. 'Scarlet fever, ma'am. Ought to have called me before,' he said crossly. Then he told me to go home and take belladonna right away or I'd have the fever."

Jo said gravely, "You've been with the baby every day for more than a week, so I'm afraid you are going to have the fever, Beth. I'll call Hannah, she knows all about sickness."

"Now I'll tell you what we'll do," said Hannah, when she had examined and questioned Beth.

"We will have Dr Bangs just to take a look at you, dear, and see that we start right," said Hannah.

Beth did have the fever and was much sicker than anyone expected.

Hannah wouldn't hear of "Mrs March bein' told and worried." She said, "We oughter send Amy off to Aunt March's for a spell, to keep her out of harm's way," as Amy had never had the fever.

Laurie found Amy sobbing with her head in the sofa cushions. "I don't wish to be sent off as if I was in the way," she began.

"Bless your heart, child, it's to keep you well. You don't want to be sick, do you?" said Laurie.

"But it's dull at Aunt March's, and she is so cross," said Amy, looking rather frightened.

"It won't be dull with me popping in every day to tell you how Beth is, and take you out gallivanting," said Laurie. "The old lady likes me, so she won't peck at us, whatever we do."

"Well – I guess I will go," said Amy slowly. So Amy departed in great state, with Jo and Laurie as escort.

Aunt March received Jo, Laurie and Amy with her usual hospitality. "What do you want now?" she asked, looking sharply over her spectacles.

Polly, the parrot, sitting on the back of her chair, called out, "Go away. No boys allowed here."

Laurie retired to the window, and Jo told Aunt March about Beth catching scarlet fever from the Hummels.

"No more than I expected, if you are allowed to go poking about among poor folks," said Aunt March. "Amy can stay and make herself useful if she isn't sick. Don't cry, child, it worries me to hear people sniff."

Amy was on the point of crying. Laurie slyly pulled the parrot's tail, which caused Polly to utter an astonished croak and call out, "Bless my boots!" in such a funny way that Amy laughed instead.

"What do you hear from your mother?" asked the old lady gruffly.

"Father is much better," replied Jo, trying to keep sober.

"Oh, is he? Well, that won't last long, I fancy. March never had any stamina," was the cheerful reply.

"Ha, ha! Never say die, take a pinch of snuff, goodbye, goodbye!" squalled Polly, dancing on his perch, and clawing at the old lady's cap as Laurie tweaked him in the rear.

"Hold your tongue, you disrespectful old bird!" exclaimed Aunt March. "And, Jo, you'd better go at once. It isn't proper to be gadding about so late with a rattlepated boy like…"

"Hold your tongue, you disrespectful old bird!" cried Polly, tumbling off the chair with a bounce, and running to peck the 'rattlepated' boy, who was shaking with laughter at the last speech.

"I don't think I can bear it, but I'll try," thought Amy, as she was left alone with Aunt March.

"Get along, you fright!" screamed Polly, and at that rude speech Amy could not restrain a sniff.

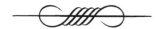

A TELEGRAM:
CHAPTER SUMMARY

A telegram informs Mrs March that Mr March, an army chaplain, is very ill in Washington. While Mrs March is in Washington nursing him, Beth falls very ill with scarlet fever. So that Amy does not catch the fever, she is sent away to stay with Aunt March.

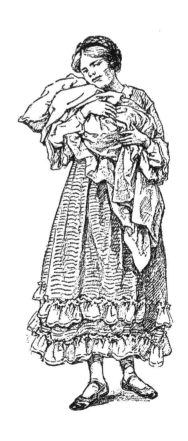

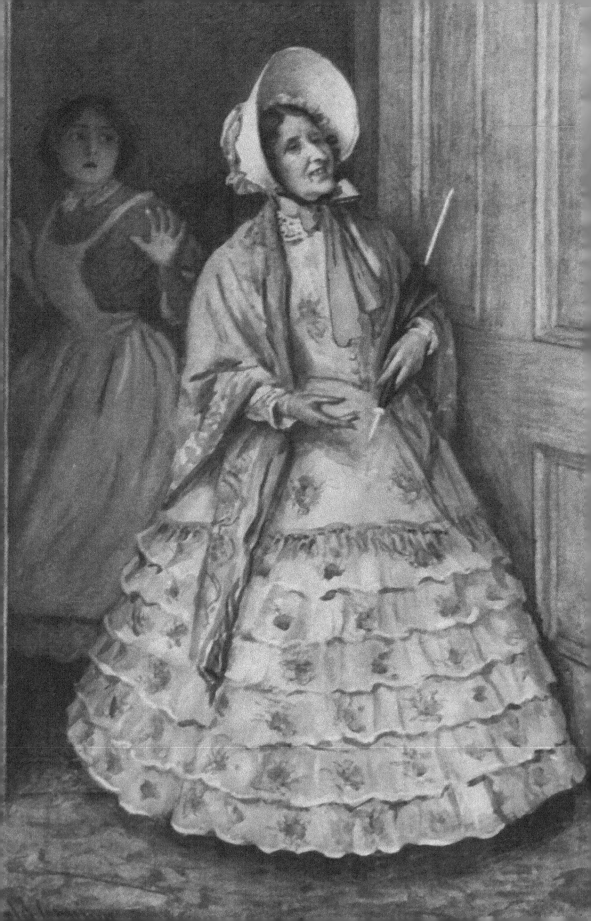

CHAPTER 5: AUNT MARCH SETTLES THE QUESTION

At old Mr Laurence's request, John Brooke, Laurie's tutor, escorted Mr and Mrs March home safely from Washington. On the return of Mr March, his wife and daughters hovered about him, neglecting everything in order to look at, wait upon, and listen to the new invalid.

Nothing seemed needed to complete the family's happiness, yet something was needed and the elder ones felt it.

Mr and Mrs March looked at one another with an anxious expression as their eyes followed Meg. Meg and John Brooke had become close. Meg was no longer herself, but now absent-minded, shy, and silent. She colored when John's name was mentioned.

Fearing that her beloved Meg might marry Mr Brooke, Jo took a dislike to him and was seen to shake her fist at his umbrella, which had been left in the hall.

Jo said to Meg, "You are not like your old self a bit, and seem ever so far away from me. I do wish it was all settled. I hate to wait. If you ever mean to marry John Brooke, make haste and have it over quickly."

"I can't say anything till he speaks," began Meg. "But if he did, I know just what I should say. I should merely say, quite calmly and decidedly, 'Thank you, Mr Brooke, you are very kind. But I agree with Father that I am too young to enter into any engagement at present. So please say no more. Let us be friends as we were.'"

Meg rose as she spoke. She was just going to rehearse the dignified exit, when a step in the hall made her fly into her seat. She began to sew as fast as if her life depended it.

Jo smothered a laugh at the sudden change. When someone gave a tap at the door, she opened it with a grim aspect which was anything but hospitable.

It was Mr Brooke, who said, "Good afternoon. I came to get my umbrella, that is, to see how your father finds himself today."

"I'll tell him you are here." Jo slipped out of the room, pleased to give Meg a chance to make her speech of polite refusal to Mr Brooke.

Meg also tried to escape, but Mr Brooke said, "Don't go. Are you afraid of me, Margaret?" He looked so hurt that Meg thought she must have done something very rude.

She answered, "How can I be afraid when you have been so kind to Father? I only wish I could thank you for it."

"Shall I tell you how?" asked Mr Brooke, holding her small hands fast in his own. "I only want to know if you care for me a little, Meg. I love you so much, dear," he added tenderly.

This was the moment for the calm, proper speech, but Meg didn't make it. She forgot every word of it, hung her head, and answered, "I don't know."

Mr Brooke said, "I'll wait, and in the meantime, you could be learning to like me. Would it be a very hard lesson, dear?"

His tone was properly beseeching. But Meg saw that his eyes were merry as well as tender, and that he wore the satisfied smile of one who had no doubt of his success. This nettled her.

She felt excited and strange, and not knowing what else to do, followed a capricious impulse. Withdrawing her hands, she said petulantly, "Perhaps learning to like you would be too hard. Please go away and let me be!"

Poor Mr Brooke looked as if his lovely castle in the air was tumbling about his ears. "Do you really mean that?" he asked anxiously.

What would have happened next I cannot say, if Aunt March had not come hobbling in at this interesting minute.

"Bless me, what's all this?" cried the old lady with a rap of her cane as she glanced from the pale young gentleman to the scarlet young lady. Mr Brooke took one look at Aunt March and vanished into the study.

"It's Mr Brooke, Father's friend. I'm so surprised to see you, Aunt March!" said Meg.

"That's evident," returned Aunt March, sitting down. "But what is Father's friend saying to make you look like a peony? There's mischief going on, and I insist upon knowing what it is!"

"Mr Brooke came for his umbrella," began Meg, wishing that Mr Brooke and the umbrella were safely out of the house.

"Brooke? The Laurence boy's tutor? Ah! I understand now. I know all about it. You haven't gone and accepted his proposal, child?" cried Aunt March, looking scandalized. "For if you mean to marry this Cook, not one penny of my money ever goes to you. Remember that, girl!" said the old lady impressively.

Now Meg was the gentlest person, but being peremptorily ordered not to marry John Brooke had the effect of immediately making up her mind that she would marry him.

With unusual spirit Meg said with a resolute air, "I shall marry whom I please, Aunt March, and you can leave your money to anyone you like."

"Highty-tighty!" said Aunt March. "Is that the way you take my advice, Miss? You'll be sorry for it by-and-by, when you've tried love in a cottage and found it a failure."

"It can't be a worse one than some people find in big houses," retorted Meg.

Aunt March took no notice, but went on with her lecture. "This Rook is poor and hasn't got any rich relations, has he?"

"No, but he has many warm friends."

"You can't live on friends, try it and see how cool they'll grow," said Aunt March. "I thought you had more sense, Meg. He knows you have got rich relations, child. That's the secret of his liking, I suspect."

"Aunt March, how dare you say such a thing?" cried Meg indignantly. "My John wouldn't marry for money, any more than I would. I'm not afraid of being poor, for I've been happy so far, and I know I shall be with him because he loves me, and I…"

Meg stopped there, remembering all of a sudden that she hadn't made up her mind, and she had told 'her John' to go away.

Aunt March was very angry, for she had set her heart on having her pretty niece make a fine match. Something in the girl's happy young face made the lonely old woman feel both sad and sour. Slamming the door in Meg's face, she drove off in high dudgeon.

Left alone, Meg stood for a moment, undecided whether to laugh or cry.

Before she could make up her mind, Mr Brooke rushed into the parlor and said all in one breath, "I couldn't help hearing, Meg. Thank you for defending me. So I needn't go away, but may stay and be happy, may I, dear?"

And Meg replied, "Yes John," and hid her face in Mr Brooke's waistcoat.

Fifteen minutes later Jo returned, expecting that her strong-minded sister Meg would by now have banished the objectionable Mr Brooke.

Jo was transfixed by the sight of the said Brooke serenely sitting on the sofa with the strong-minded sister enthroned upon his knee and wearing an expression of abject submission.

It was altogether too much for Jo. She rushed upstairs to find her parents and cried, "Oh, do somebody go down quick! John Brooke is acting dreadfully, and Meg likes it!"

But when John Brooke described for the family the paradise he meant to earn for Meg, and when he took her into supper, both looked so happy that Jo hadn't the heart to be jealous or dismal.

Amy was very much impressed by John's devotion and Meg's dignity. Beth beamed at them from a distance. And Mr and Mrs March surveyed the young couple with tender satisfaction.

No one ate much, but everyone looked very happy. The old room seemed to have brightened up amazingly when the first romance of the family began there.

Mrs March said, "The joys come close upon the sorrows this time, and I rather think the changes for the better have begun. In most families there comes, now and then, a year full of events. This has been such a one, but it ends well, after all."

Then Laurie came prancing in, overflowing with good spirits, bearing a great bridal-looking bouquet for Meg. He evidently labored under the delusion that the whole marriage proposal and acceptance had been brought about by his excellent management.

As Jo's eyes went slowly round the room, they brightened as they looked, for the prospect was a pleasant one.

Father and Mother sat together, quietly reliving the first chapter of the romance, which for them began some twenty years ago. Amy was drawing the lovers, who sat apart in a beautiful world of their own, the light of which touched their faces with a grace the little artist could not copy.

Beth lay on her sofa, talking cheerily with old Mr
Laurence. The old man held her little hand as if he
felt that it possessed the power to lead him along
the peaceful way she walked.

Jo lounged in her favorite low seat, with the grave
quiet look which best became her. Laurie leaned on
the back of her chair, his chin on a level with her
curly head and smiled with his friendliest aspect.

So the curtain falls upon Meg, Jo, Beth, and Amy.
Whether it ever rises again, depends upon the
reception given the first act of the domestic drama
called Little Women.

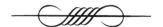

AUNT MARCH SETTLES THE QUESTION:
CHAPTER SUMMARY

Mr March returns home, and Mr Brooke proposes
to Meg. Jo fears losing Meg but on seeing how
happy the lovers are, she warms to the idea.
Aunt March disapproves of the match because
Brooke is not rich, but Meg stands her ground.

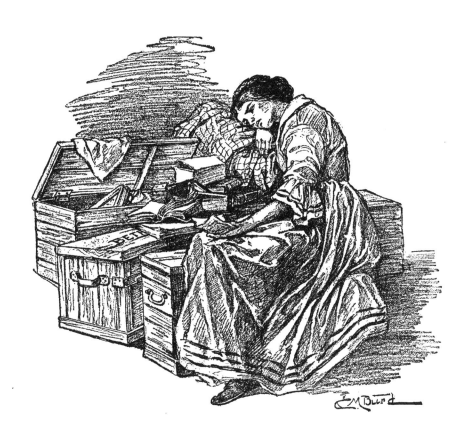

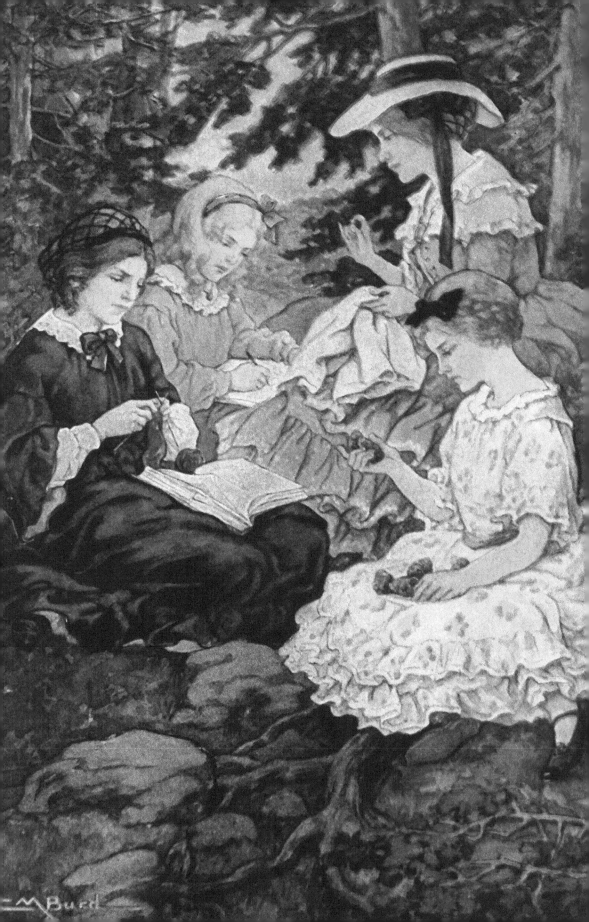